KETO
DIET FOR
BEGINNERS

The Keto Diet Cookbook with Quick and Healthy
Recipes incl. 30 Days Weight Loss Challenge

1st Edition

Sarah Amber Patterson

ISBN- 9781093841909

TABLE OF CONTENTS

EXCLUSIVE BONUS!

Get Keto Audiobook for FREE NOW!*

*The Ultimate Keto Diet Guide 2019-2020:
How to Loose weight with Quick and Easy Steps*

SCAN ME

or go to

www.free-keto.co.uk

*Listen free for 30 Days on Audible (for new members only)

INTRODUCTION

The popularity of the ketogenic diet has reached unexpected levels over the past few years even though its principles go against the widespread misconception that fats are responsible for the obesity epidemics that has spread across the glove. So, what makes so many people embrace not only a low-carb diet, but a high fat one? And what is the secret of a successful keto diet? This book is all about explaining the keto diet and how you can secure its benefits for long-term health and weight loss.

What is Keto?

In short, keto is a high-fat, low-carb diet. In order to understand how the ketogenic diet works, you must first understand what happens in your body when you eat a typical high-carb, low fat diet. Carbs are the body's main source of energy. The body converts carbs into glucose and uses it as immediate fuel its various processes. In addition, it converts some of the carbs into glycogen and stores it for future use. However, in a high-carb diet, the body ends up with more carbs that it needs for immediate use and more carbs that it can store for future use. What does the body do with all the additional carbs? Unfortunately, it converts the extra carbs into fat.

By reducing the amount of carbs, the keto dieter forces the body to use the next available source to produce energy, i.e., fats. Hence, the body turns to fats as its primary source of energy. It starts breaking down fats into ketones and uses them as fuel. The process is called ketosis and it is the exact opposite of the body's natural metabolic tendency.

Keto is a low-carbohydrate, adequate protein, and high-fat diet. The largest part of the calories will, therefore, come from fats rather than carbs. The ketogenic diet is embraced by those who eat animal-based diets, as well as those who eat plant-based diets.

Keto dieters can turn to high-fat animal products, such as butter, meats, and full-fat dairy. However, vegans can also follow a keto diet by increasing their intake of high-fat plant-based foods, including vegetable oils, seeds, nuts, and avocados.

Did you know?

For decades, keto and low-carb diets have been used in treating epilepsy in children. There are studies that are currently focused on discovering the effects of low-carb intake on other brain conditions.

How much carbs can I eat?

The ketogenic diet is not a no-carb diet; it's a low-carb diet. But how much is too low and how much is not low enough? To put it shortly, the smaller the carb intake, the more effective the diet seems to be in fighting off anger while maintaining weight loss. The same principle applies if your aim is to reverse type 2 diabetes.

However, the fewer carbs you eat, the more challenging and restrictive the diet will feel. Below you can find three examples of a keto diet based on carb intake:

- **Strict ketogenic diet:** under 20g of carbs per day
- **Moderate keto diet:** 20-50g of carbs per day
- **Liberal keto diet:** 20-100 g of carbs per day

How much fat do you need to eat?

The body needs energy to function and there are two sources of energy available: carbohydrates and fats. Typically, the body will use carbs to convert to fuel, but, if you take the carbs away, you leave the body with fats to burn for fuel. For the body to burn fat and not carbs, you need a lower carb intake and a higher fat intake concomitantly. Obviously, most of your calories will come from fats.

The body will turn to its fat stores once it has consumed all the fat that you have provided through food. Therefore, if you want to lose weight, you need to provide the body with just enough fat to trigger ketosis and encourage weight loss. As with all diets, you must be balanced: eat enough fats to feel great and satisfied and still lose weight. Not eating enough fats on a low-carb diet will make you feel hungry or tired.

Advantages of a Keto Diet

Fats have been blamed for the obesity that seems to have plagued the world over the past two decades. However, more recent studies come to support the exact opposite. If you give the body fewer carbs and more fats, it will not have enough carbs to use for fuel. The body will have no choice but to turn to the next available source of energy: fats. The result? Fat loss.

Here are some of the most popular benefits of a keto diet:

- Reduces appetite and, automatically, calorie intake.
- Leads to abdominal fat loss, which is responsible for metabolic problems.
- Reduces blood triglycerides, responsible for increased risk heart disease.

- Increases the levels of HDL cholesterol (the good cholesterol) and reduces the levels of LDL cholesterol (the bad cholesterol).
- Stabilizes blood sugar levels and reduces insulin levels.
- Lower blood pressure reducing risk of cardiac disease complications.
- Minimizes the symptoms of metabolic syndrome, known for increasing the risk of Type 2 diabetes and heart disease.

What to Eat in a Keto Diet?

The ketogenic diet is simply defined as a low-carb, high-fat diet. But how does that translate into actual eating habits? What foods are you allowed to eat and what is prohibited on a keto diet? Let's start with the categories of foods that are essential in a keto diet:

Meats

It is preferable to eat unprocessed meats that come from grass-fed animals and organic farms. If you do eat processed meats, make sure they contain under 5% carbs. As far as the quantity, you must stick to a normal intake. Meats are high-protein foods and, if you eat too much meat, you will get excess protein, which is not compatible with a keto diet. The body will convert the additional protein and not the fat, into glucose and fuel the body. This can cancel completely or at least reduce ketosis, the very essence of a ketogenic diet.

Fish and seafood

There are no restrictions as far as this category of foods is concerned. Fatty fish is particularly popular in a ketogenic lifestyle. Salmon, mackerel, or tuna are great options. Of course, wild-caught fish is always the best option since breading fish will be higher in carbs.

Eggs

Eggs are one of the most popular foods in a ketogenic diet. You can cook them to your preference and eat them at breakfast, lunch, or dinner. Eggs are extremely versatile in recipes and can be adapted to suit almost any taste. Try to stick to healthy options, such as free-range and organic eggs. As far as quantity is concerned, 3-6 eggs per day is a healthy intake.

Fruits

Moderation is key when it comes to fruits in a keto diet. Remember that the carbs in fruits are mostly sugars. Low-carb fruits are compatible with a keto diet. Berries, melons, stone fruits, avocados, and tomatoes are some of the most popular choices due to their low-carb content. Apples and bananas, on the other hand, are high in carbs, and less compatible with a keto diet. You can integrate fruits in your diet successfully if you stick to your target carb intake. However, to make it easier to stay away from fruits think of them as natural candy. No matter how you look at it, fruit is sugar.

Non-starchy Veggies

You can consume vegetables growing above the ground, i.e., non-starchy vegetables, fresh or frozen. Leafy greens are particularly popular. Favourite choices include cabbage, green beans, cauliflower, broccoli, and zucchini. Versatile, flavourful, and colourful, vegetables that grow above the ground are excellent choices for keto dieters.

You can cook them any way you like them. Considering that keto is all about a high-fat intake, you can add extra flavour to your veggies because you can fry them in generous amounts of oil or butter. In fact, keto dieters eat a lot more veggies that other dieters considering that veggies basically replace what used to be staple foods: pasta, potatoes, and rice.

High-fat Dairy

So many people that go for a keto diet choose it because they can finally eat all those tasty high-fat dairy products. In fact, lighter versions, or diet versions, contain a lot of added sugar, i.e., carbs. Favourites include full-fat cheese and butter. A moderate amount of high-fat yogurt is fine, but don't overdo it.

However, milk must be consumed sparingly. Remember that a latte has 18 g of carbs while a glass of milk is packed with 15 g of carbs. Just remember that a high-fat diet doesn't mean free hand at snacking on cheese when not hungry. It's a high fat diet, not an excess fat diet.

Nuts

Nuts are great sources of healthy fats and are very compatible with a keto diet. However, snacking on nuts is not a smart idea. First, it's very easy to eat nuts in excess because they are incredibly tasty. The best way to incorporate nuts in your keto diet is to have them sprinkled on salads. Also, not all nuts are low-carb so stick to whole nuts, pecans, macadamia nuts, rather than cashew nuts. Again, you must remember that the ketogenic diet is not about eating fats in excess. It's about eating more fat than carbs to trigger ketosis and generate weight loss.

Drinks

- **Water**

You and enjoy water with ice, plain, or sparkling. You can flavour it with limes, lemons, mint or cucumbers. Add a touch of salt to your water if you experience keto flu symptoms

- **Unsweetened coffee**

It is preferable you have your coffee black, but you can add a little cream or milk. Unless you drink 5 large coffees every day, you should be fine. You can fortify your coffee with coconut oil or MCT oil and butter and get a bulletproof coffee.

- **Unsweetened tea**

Keto dieters can consume tea freely, no matter which type of tea they prefer. However, stay away from the typical English black tea because the milk in it will ruin your low-carb effort. And, of course, you can only have your tea without sugar.

- **Bone broth**

Simple to make, bone broth is satisfying, packed with electrolytes and nutrients, and very hydrating. You are welcome to make your own bone broth and you can always fortify it with a touch of butter.

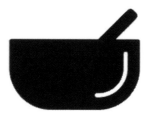

What NOT to Eat in a Keto Diet?

Sugar

The keto diet is not a very restrictive diet but there are a couple of absolute no-nos. Sugar is the big no-no for the keto diet. Essentially, no sugar translates into no fruit juice, no soft drinks, no vitamin water, no sports drinks. Next, you must avoid another category of sugar-packed foods: sweets, homemade or processed, it doesn't matter. Keto says no to cakes, candy, cookies, donuts, chocolate bars, frozen treats, or breakfast cereals.

Tip! Always read all labels since sugars can be a hidden ingredient in the foods you least expect it! Check labels for drinks, condiments, sauces, dressings or any other packaged goods. As a rule, stay away from any sweeteners, including "healthy" agave syrup, maple syrup, or honey, and artificial sweeteners.

Starch

Another no-no in the keto diet is starch. There are so many sources of starch that you really must pay extra attention. The obvious are pasta, bread, pasta, and rice, muesli – wholegrain or not. Legumes are also high-carb, especially beans and lentils. Some root vegetables, such as celery root, are acceptable in small amounts.

However, there are keto versions of some of these high-carb foods, such as keto pasta, keto rice, keto breads, etc.

Drinks

Beer is an absolute no-no because it's nothing but liquid bread. It is packed with rapid-absorption carbohydrates. If you really must have a beer, try a lower-carb one.

Margarine

With a very high omega-6 content, margarine is a heavily processed product and believed to be linked to a variety of inflammatory diseases, including allergies and asthma. It is preferable that you avoid margarine all together since your diet allows for the use of quality high-fat dairy, such as butter or olive oil.

How to start with a Keto Diet?

A low-carb diet essentially translates into a diet that is low on starches and sugars. Ac smaller starch and sugar intake allows for blood sugar levels to stabilize and insulin levels to drop since you don't need high levels of insulin to control blood sugar levels. Remember insulin is also called the fat-storing hormone. A lower insulin level increases the fat burning process and for the feeling of satiety (fullness) to install quicker. Since you feel full quicker, you will eat less. Eating less leads to weight loss.

However, you must be aware that the body is not used to burning fat for fuel. The body is used to having enough carbs available to convert to glucose and then energy. The body is addicted to carbs. The drastic drop in carb levels will cause the body to enter withdrawal. Carb withdrawal symptoms mimic flu symptoms, which is why it's often referred to as the keto flu. The keto flu lasts, in most cases, no more than a week, but some keto dieters have experienced the symptoms for periods longer than that.

Not all people experience the keto flu, but you should be prepared to deal with them in case you do. Keto flu symptoms include nausea, vomiting, headaches, constipation/diarrhoea, irritability, muscle cramps and weakness, dizziness or poor concentration, and even stomach pain. Some complain about having difficulty sleeping while many experience sugar cravings.

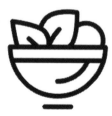

Recipes for Breakfast

Cottage cheese pancakes with berries

Time: 15 minutes | Serves: 4
Net carbs: 5 g
Fibre: 3 g
Fat: 39 g
Protein: 13 g
Kcal: 425

Ingredients:

- 4 eggs
- 200 gr cottage cheese
- 1 tbsp psyllium husk powder (ground)
- 60 gr coconut oil or butter

For serving:

- 1 cup heavy whipping cream
- ½ cup fresh berries (raspberries, blueberries, or strawberries)

Preparation:

1. In a medium-size mixing bowl, combine the cottage cheese, eggs, and psyllium husk powder. Allow 5 to 10 minutes for the mixture to thicken.
2. In a non-stick skillet, heat up the coconut oil or butter on low to medium heat.
3. Fry each pancake for 3 to 4 minutes on each side. Keep them to a size that allows for easy flipping.
4. In a separate bowl, whisk the whipping cream until it forms soft peaks.
5. Top the pancakes with whipped cream and serve with desired berries.

Classic bacon and eggs

Time: 15 minutes | Serves: 4
Net carbs: 1 g
Fibre: 3 g
Fat: 22 g
Protein: 15 g
Kcal: 272

Ingredients:

- ♦   140 gr bacon rashers
- ♦   8 eggs

Optional:

- ♦   Cherry tomatoes
- ♦   Fresh parsley

Preparation:

1. Placea pan over medium heat and fry the bacon until it becomes crispy. Set aside on a plate. Keep the bacon grease in the pan.
2. Crackthe eggs in therendered grease and fry them over medium heat. Cook the eggs to desired consistency.
3. While the eggs are cooking, cutthe cherry tomatoes in half and add them to the pan. Cook to your preference.
4. Season with salt and pepper. Serve with fresh parsley!

Buttery coconut flour waffles

Time: 30 minutes | Serves: 5
Net carbs: 4 g
Fibre: 3 g
Fat: 26 g
Protein: 8 g
Kcal: 278

Ingredients:

- 5 eggs whites
- 5 egg yolks
- 4 tbsp granulated stevia
- 4 tbsp coconut flour
- 1 tsp baking powder
- 3 tbsp full-fat milk
- 2 tsp vanilla extract
- 1/2 cup melted butter

Preparation:

1. Place the egg yolks in bowl and gently mix with the stevia, baking powder, and coconut flower.
2. Fold the butter in the mixture until it forms a smooth batter.
3. Incorporate the vanilla extract and milk into the mixture.
4. Place the egg whites into a separate bowl and whisk until fluffy.
5. Spoon by spoon, fold in the fluffy egg whites into the flour and butter mixture.
6. In a hot waffle maker, pour the resulting mixture. Cook the waffles to the desired color. Enjoy!

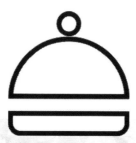

15-min creamy seafood omelette

Time: 15 minutes | Serves: 2
Net carbs: 4 g
Fibre: 1 g
Fat: 83 g
Protein: 27 g
Kcal: 872

Ingredients:

- 150 gr cooked shrimp
- 2 tbsp olive oil
- 1red chili pepper
- ½ cup mayonnaise
- ½tsp ground cumin

- 1 tbsp chives (fresh or dried)
- 2 tbsp olive oil orbutter
- 6 eggs
- salt and pepper

Optional:

- 2 garlic cloves

Preparation:

1. Preheat broiler.
2. Place the shrimp in a bowl and mix with the olive oil, ground cumin, chilli pepper, salt and pepper, and minced garlic (optional). Broil the shrimp and set aside to cool.
3. Once the shrimp mixture has cooled, add the chives and mayo and mix.
4. In a mixing bowl, whisk the eggs and add salt and pepper to taste. Whisk the eggs together. Season with salt and pepper. Fry in a non-stick skillet with plenty of butter or oil.
5. Add oil or butter to a non-stick skillet. Pour the egg mixture and let the eggs fry on medium heat.
6. When nearly done, place the shrimp mixture on one half of theomelette. Fold the other half over and allow the omelette to set completely on low heat. Serve hot.

Smoked salmon and scrambled eggs sandwich

Time: 15 minutes | Serves: 4
Net carbs: 3 g
Fibre: 4 g
Fat: 55 g
Protein: 41g
Kcal: 678

Ingredients:

- 4 eggs
- 2 tablespoons double cream
- 2 tablespoons salted butter at room temperature
- 100 gr smoked salmon
- 1 pinch chili flakes
- 30 gr lettuce leaves or rocket leaves
- salt and pepper
- 2slices of low-carb bread (keto pumpkin bread)
- 50 gr butter for frying

Optional:

- 1 tbsp fresh chives

Preparation:

1. In a mixing bowl, whisk the whipping cream, eggs, and chilli flakes together and season with salt and pepper.
2. Placethe butter in anon-stick skillet and allow to melt on medium heat. Pour the cream and egg mixture into the hot butter. Stir until cooked through. Remove from heat.
3. Take two slices of low-carb bread and toast them. Spread the butter in a thick layer on each slice.
4. Place the lettuce (rocket) leaves on each slice. Gently place the scrambled eggs on the green leaves and top with the salmon. Decorate with finely chopped chives.

Guacamole and bacon breakfast tacos

Time: 15 minutes | Serves: 2
Net carbs: 4 g
Fibre: 5 g
Fat: 35 g
Protein: 11 g
Kcal: 387

Ingredients:

- 2 eggs (free-range)
- 1 tbsp Brain Octane oil
- 1 avocado (medium)
- 1 tbsp ghee

- 1/4 tspHimalayan salt (pink)
- 2 rashers unsmoked bacon (cooked)
- 1/4 cupromaine lettuce (chopped)
- 3 tbsp diced sweet potatoes (cooked)

Optional:

- Finely chopped coriander

Preparation:

1. Heat the ghee in a small frying pan over medium heat.
2. **For the taco shells:** crack one egg into the centre of the pan. Pierce the yolk and allow to cook for 1-2 minutes on each side. Remove from pan and place on a plate lined with baking paper.Repeat for the remainingegg.
3. Place avocado, oil, and salt in a small bowl and mash to the desired consistency.
4. **For serving:** Spread half of the octane oil and avocado mixture on each taco (egg) shell. Top the avocado shells with lettuce, one slice of bacon, and sweet potatoes. Sprinkle chopped coriander and season with Himalayan pink salt. Fold and enjoy!

Brussels Sprouts Hash

Time: 20 minutes | Serves: 4
Net carbs: 3 g
Fibre: 4 g
Fat: 55 g
Protein: 41g
Kcal: 678

Ingredients:

- 6 bacon rashers
- 500 gr brussels sprouts (trimmed and quartered)
- 1/2 yellow onion (chopped)
- Salt and ground black pepper
- 2 garlic cloves (minced)
- 1/4tspred pepper flakes
- 4 large free-range eggs
- 3 tbsp water

Preparation:

5. Cut the bacon rashers into 1" pieces. Placein a frying pan and fry over medium heat until crispy. Turn off the heat and remove bacon.Place on plate lined with paper-towel. Keep the bacon fat but remove any black bits.

6. Add the chopped onion and brussels sprouts to the bacon fat and cook on medium heat stirring occasionally until the vegetables turn golden and start to soften. Sprinkle in the red pepper flakes, salt, and ground pepper and season to taste.

7. Add the water and place a lid over the frying pan. Continue to cook for five more minutes until the water has nearly evaporated and the sprouts are tender. Addthe minced garlic and allow to cook for another minute until fragrant.

8. Create four holes in the sprouts and onion hash. Crack one egg in each hole. Sprinkle with salt and pepper and cover the pan. Allow to cook until the eggs are cooked to the desired consistency.

9. Top with the crispy bacon bits. Serve immediately! Enjoy!

Keto Oatmeal

Time: 30 minutes | Serves: 10
Net carbs: 9 g
Fibre: 8 g
Fat: 62 g
Protein: 10 g
Kcal: 621

Ingredients:

- 1 cup coconut milk
- 1 tbsp chia seeds
- 1 tbsp flaxseed
- 1 tbsp sunflower seeds
- salt

Preparation:

1. Combine the coconut milk, chia seeds, flaxseed, and sunflower seeds in a small pan. Bring the mixture to a boil.
2. Lower the heat and allow to simmer for a couple more minutes until the mixture hasreached the preferred consistency.
3. Decorate with the topping of choice: fresh berries, cinnamon, almond milk, coconut milk, or butter! Enjoy!

Low-carb turkey and avocado plate

Time: 15 minutes | Serves: 2
Net carbs: 9 g
Fibre: 4 g
Fat: 84 g
Protein: 24 g
Kcal: 820

Ingredients:

- 2 medium avocados
- 180 deli turkey
- 60 gr romaine lettuce leaves
- 90 gr softcheese (full-fat)
- 4 tbsp olive oil
- salt and pepper

Preparation:

1. Half and slice the avocados. Place the soft cheese on turkey slices and roll.
2. Arrange the sliced avocados, turkey and softcheese rolls, and lettuce leaves on a plate.
3. Sprinkle the lettuce and avocados with the olive oil. Season with salt and pepper. Enjoy!

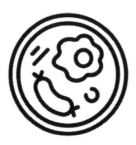

Spinach frittata keto-style

Time: 15 minutes | Serves: 2
Net carbs: 9 g
Fibre: 4 g
Fat: 84 g
Protein: 24 g
Kcal: 820

Ingredients:

- 150 diced bacon
- or
- 150 diced chorizo sausage
- 8 free-range eggs

- 220 gr fresh baby spinach
- 1 cup double cream
- 150 grated cheddar cheese
- salt and pepper

For frying:

- 2 tbsp salted butter

Preparation:

1. Pre-heat oven to 175°C (350°F)
2. Placea frying pan over medium heat andmelt the butter. Add the diced bacon (chorizo) and fry until crispy. Add the spinach. Cook until spinach has wilted, stirring occasionally. Remove from heat.
3. Whisk double cream and egg together until combined.Pour mixture into a 9x9" (22 x 22 cm) baking tray that has been previously greased. Top with the spinach, bacon, and cheese.
4. Place the oven tray in the middle of the oven. Allow to bake until golden brown on top and set in the middle (25-30 minutes). Cut into squares and serve immediately!

Recipes for Lunch

Bun-less cheeseburgers

Time: 20 minutes | Serves: 6
Net carbs: 4 g
Fibre: 1.8 g
Fat: 22.8 g
Protein: 29.1 g
Kcal: 336/cheeseburger

Ingredients:

- 500gr 20% fat mince beef
- 1 tsp pinkHimalayan salt
- 1tbsp Worcestershire sauce
- 1 tbsp avocado oil

- 6 slices mature cheddar cheese
- 12 portobello mushroom caps
- 1 tsp black pepper

Optional:

- Romaine lettuce
- Fried onions
- Dill pickles

- Keto mustard
- Keto barbecue sauce

Preparation:

1. Combine the groundbeefwith salt, pepper, and Worcestershire sauce in a bowl. Shape the beef mixture into six burger patties.
2. Place a large frying pan over medium heat and add the avocado oil. Add the mushroom caps and let cook for 3 to 4 minutes on each side. Remove from pan and set aside.
3. Place the burger patties in the same pan. Allow them to cook the patties until desired doneness. Top the patties withthe cheese slices. Cover the pan and allow 1 minute for the cheddar cheese to melt.
4. Assemble the layers of the portobello mushroom burgers: Portobello mushroom cap, cheeseburger, garnish of choice, portobello mushroom cap.
5. Serve immediately! Enjoy!

Keto curried chicken "wraps"

Time: 20 minutes | Serves: 2
Net carbs: 7.4 g
Fibre: 0 g
Fat: 36.4 g
Protein: 50.9 g
Kcal: 554

Ingredients:

- 500 gr boneless thigh fillets
- 2 minced garlic cloves
- 1/4 cup minced onion
- 2 tsp Red Madrascurry powder
- 1tspblack pepper
- 1.5 tsp pink Himalayansalt

- 1 cupcauliflower rice
- 3tbsp pure butter ghee
- 1/4 cup coconut milkyogurt, unsweetened
- 8 small lettuce leaves

Preparation:

1. Cut the chicken thighs into 1" pieces.
2. Prepare the cauliflower rice. Arrange the lettuce wraps on a plate.
3. Place 2 tbsp of ghee in a large frying pan and heat on medium heat. Add the onions and cook while stirring until brown.
4. Add the garlic, sliced chicken, and salt to the pan and stir well. Allow to brownfor about 8 minutes.
5. Incorporate the curry powder, remaining ghee, and cauliflower rice. Sauté all ingredients until well combined.
6. Spoon the chicken curry into each lettuce wrap. Serve with coconut milk yogurt!

Pesto salmon

Time: 25 minutes | Serves: 4
Net carbs: 3 g
Fibre: 0 g
Fat: 90 g
Protein: 49 g
Kcal: 1030

Ingredients:

- 120 g green pesto, divided
- 900 g salmon
- salt and pepper

- ½ cup Greek yogurt
- 1 cup mayonnaise

Preparation:

1. Pre-heat oven at 200°C (400°F).
2. Grease an oven tray. Place the salmon fillets skin-side down in the baking tray. Sprinkle salt and pepper to taste and cost lightly with half the pesto.
3. Place the oven tray with the salmon fillets in the oven and bake for 30 minutes. The salmonshould flake easily when done.
4. Prepare the green sauce my combining the remaining ingredients: yogurt, mayonnaise, and pesto.
5. Grease an oven tray. Place the salmon fillets skin-side down in the baking tray. Sprinkle salt and pepper to taste and cost lightly with pesto. Serve with simple sides, such as steamed broccoli or an energy-packed salad of pecans, greens, seeds, and a drizzle of homemade vinaigrette.

Cream-cheese keto turkey

Time: 50 minutes | Serves: 4
Net carbs: 7 g
Fibre: 0 g
Fat: 67 g
Protein: 43 g
Kcal: 593

Ingredients:

- 4 medium turkey breast fillets
- 2 cups crème fraiche
- 2 tbsp butter
- 200 g soft cheese (cream cheese)
- salt and pepper
- 1/3 cupcapers (small variety)

Preparation:

1. Pre-heat oven to 180°C (360°F).
2. Place one tbsp of butter in a baking pan and allow to melt over medium heat. Season the turkey breasts with salt and pepper. Place in the baking pan and let fry on both sides until golden brown.
3. Remove the pan from heat and place in the oven. Allow the turkey breasts to cook through. Remove from oven and place the breasts on aplate. Tent with foil.
4. In a small sauce pan, combine turkey drippings, sour cream, and soft cheese. Gently bring to a boil while stirring. Season with salt and pepper and reduce heat. Allow the sauce to simmer until the desired thickness.
5. In a frying pan, place remaining butter and melt over high heat. Add the capers and sauté until crispy.
6. Slice the turkey breasts and drizzle generously with the sauce. Top with the fried capers. Sides include broccoli or cauliflower mash.

Creamy cabbage with fried chorizo

Time: 30 minutes | Serves: 2
Net carbs: 6 g
Fibre: 0 g
Fat: 66 g
Protein: 23.5 g
Kcal: 730

Ingredients:

- 350 g chorizo sausage
- 1 tbsp butter
- Creamed cabbage
- 30 g butter
- 350 g green cabbage

- ¾ cup double cream
- ¼ cup finely chopped fresh parsley
- salt and pepper
- zest of ¼ lemon

Preparation:

1. Placethe butter in a non-stick frying pan andallow to melt over medium heat. Add the chorizo sausage and fry until desired doneness. Remove from pan and place in an air tightcontainerto keep warm.
2. Use a food processor orsharp knife toshred the green cabbage.
3. Add the remaining butter to the chorizo fat in the same pan.Add the shreddedcabbage and sauté cabbage over medium heat until golden brown. Stir occasionally.
4. Add double cream to the cabbage hash and bring to a gentle boil. Lower the heat and allow for the cream to reduce until the desired thickness.Sprinkle salt and pepper to taste and garnish with lemon zest and chopped parsley.
5. Serve the chorizo with the creamy cabbage and the green salad of choice.

Avocado and green beans pork chops

Ingredients:

- 4 pork shoulder chops
- 2 tbsp olive oil
- 2 tbspchipotle paste (mild)
- ½ tsp salt
- 125 g butter at room temperature
- ½ tsp salt
- 1 garlic clove
- ¼ tsp paprika powder
- ¼tsp ground black pepper

- 2 tbspolive oil
- 280 g green beans (fresh)
- ½tsp salt
- ¼ tsp ground black pepper
- 6 green onionssprings (scallions)
- 2 medium avocados
- fresh parsley (optional)
- pepper to taste

Preparation:

1. **Pork shoulder chops:** In a small bowl, mix the oil, chipotle paste, and salt. Brush the pork chops with the mixture. Allow 15 minutes to marinate.
2. Pre-heat oven to 200°C (400°F). Place a rack on an oven tray or baking paper and grill the marinated meat 10-15 minutes on each side or until the meat is done.
3. **Garlic butter:** mix garlic with spices and butter and let sit.
4. **Green beans and avocado:** Pour the oil in a medium frying panandheat on medium high. Add the green beans and sauté for 4 minutes. Reduce heat, add spices, and cook for another minute until the beanshave turned a nice colour.
5. Mash the avocados to a smooth consistency with a fork. Added the finely sliced green onions and combine. Add the avocado and scallion mixture into the green beans. Sprinkle on pepper to taste and decorate with finely chopped parsley.

One-pot kale and bacon

Time: 15 minutes | Serves: 2
Net carbs: 13 g
Fibre: 3 g
Fat: 90 g
Protein: 55 g
Kcal: 980

Ingredients:

- 300g pre-washed baby kale
- 170g diced smoked bacon
- 4 eggs
- 75 g butter
- 30g pecan nuts
- ¼ cup frozen cranberries (or other berries)
- salt and pepper

Preparation:

1. Heat ⅔ of the butter in a frying pan over medium heat. Add the baby kaleand increase the heat to high. Fry the kale until edges turn slightly brown. Remove from pan and set aside.
2. In the same pan, add the diced bacon and sear until crispy. Lower the heat and return the wilted kale to the pan. Add the frozen cranberries and pecan nuts. Stir to warm through.
3. Serve immediately! Enjoy!

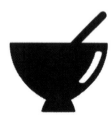

Roasted bell peppers and fried halloumi cheese

Time: 40 minutes | Serves: 4
Net carbs: 10 g
Fibre: 3 g
Fat: 99 g
Protein: 31 g
Kcal: 1061

Ingredients:

- 550 halloumi cheese (cut in 8 thick slices)
- 8 large red bell peppers
- 120 ml olive oil
- 1 tsp dried oregano

Cucumber Salad

- 160 ml mayonnaise
- 75 g soft cheese
- 60 g chopped dill pickles
- 60 g diced cucumber
- Salt and pepper
- 2 tsp dried mint

Preparation:

1. **Fried peppers:** Pre-heat the oven to 225°C (450°F). Line a baking tray with baking paper. Place the bell peppers in thetry, stems outwards. Brush the peppers with olive oil on all sides. Roast the bell peppers for 20 minutes until the skin turns a little black. Turn the bell peppers after half the time. Remove from oven and place in a paper bag in fridge for 10 minutes. Remove from paper bag and peel the bell peppers. Season with salt and pepper!
2. **Cucumber salad:** Combine all cucumbersalad ingredients in a small bowl and place infridgewhile you prepare thefried cheese.
3. **Fried cheese:** Sprinkle the cheese slices with dried oregano and coast with olive oil. Place remaining olive oil in a frying pan and fry the cheese slices for 2 minutes on each side.
4. Arrange cheese, cucumber salad, and roasted bell peppers on four plates and serve! Enjoy!

Cloud bread BLT

Time: 40 minutes | Serves: 4
Net carbs: 4 g
Fibre: 1 g
Fat: 48 g
Protein: 11 g
Kcal: 498

Ingredients:

Cloud bread

- 120 g cream cheese
- 3 eggs
- 1 pinch salt
- ½ tsp baking powder
- ½ tbsp ground psyllium husk powder
- ¼ tsp cream of tartar

Toppings

- 150 g smoked or unsmoked bacon rashers
- 8 tbsp mayonnaise
- 50 g lettuce
- 1 thinly sliced tomato

Optional:

- Fresh basil

Preparation:

1. **Cloud bread:** Pre-heat oven to 150°C (300°F).
2. Separate the yolks and egg whites in two bowls. Add a pinch of salt and cream of tartar to the egg whites bowl. Use a hand-held mixer to whisk into a stiff mixture.
3. Add soft cheese, baking powder, and psyllium seed husk to the egg yolks bowl. Mix to combine. Fold in the stiff egg whites into the cheese and egg yolks mixture.
4. Place the bread mixture in 8 pieces on a bakingtray previously lined with baking sheet. Placein the pre-heated oven and cook for 20-30 minutes. The bread should have a golden texture. Remove cloud bread from oven.

5. **The BLT:** Place bacon rashers in a frying pan and cook untilcrispy on medium heat.Remove from pan and set aside on a plate.

6. **Assemble the BLT:** Spread mayo on each piece of the top-side down cloud bread. Layer lettuce, sliced tomatoes, crispy bacon rashers, and fresh basil on four cloud breads. Topwith the remainingcloud bread pieces. Serve warm and enjoy!

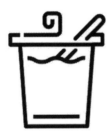

Asian-style sesame fried beef salad

Time: 40 minutes | Serves: 2
Net carbs: 7 g
Fibre: 3 g
Fat: 98 g
Protein: 34 g
Kcal: 1042

Ingredients:

Salad

- 75 g lettuce
- 50 g cucumber
- 80 g plum cherry tomatoes
- ½ red onion
- Fresh coriander or parsley
- 2 spring onion springs
- 1 tbsp (10 g) sesame seeds

Fried beef

- 300 g ribeye steaks
- 1 tbsp fish sauce
- 1 tbsp olive oil
- 1 tsp chili flakes
- 1 tbsp grated fresh ginger

Mayonnaise

- 1 tsp Dijon mustard
- 1egg yolk
- 125 ml avocado oil
- 1 tbsp sesame oil
- salt andpepper
- ½tbsp lime juice

Preparation:

1. **Marinade:** Mix olive oil, fish sauce, ginger, and chilli flakes in a plastic bag. Add the ribeye steaksand allow to marinate at room temperature for at least 20 minutes.
2. **Beef:** Remove the steaks from plastic bag and pat dry. In a medium frying pan, place the ribeye steaksand fry for1-2minutes on each side untildesired doneness.

3. **Toasted sesame seeds:** Heat a frying pan over medium heat and add the sesame seeds. Toast until fragrant and lightly browned and fragrant (2 minutes). Remove from pan and set aside.

4. **Salad:** Chop vegetables, exceptgreen onions, into bite-sized pieces and place on two plates/ salad bowls. Finely slice the green onions and set aside on aseparate plate.

5. **Sesame mayo:** Mix the egg yolk with Dijon mustard until well combined. Start pouring in very slowly the avocado oil while mixing. It's best to use and hand-held mixer for whisking. When the mayonnaise has emulsifiedalmost completely, incorporatethe sesame oil, salt and pepper, and lime juice. Continue to whisk until emulsified and reserve.

6. **Assembling:** Slice the fried ribeye steaks into thin slices and arrange on top of the chopped vegetables on plates/salad bowls. Sprinkle with the toasted sesame seeds and green onions and serve with mayonnaise.

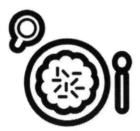

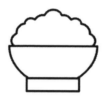

Recipes for Dinner

Hearty chicken casserole

Time: 40 minutes | Serves: 6
Net carbs: 6 g
Fibre: 2 g
Fat: 56 g
Protein: 36 g
Kcal: 675

Ingredients:

- 2 tbsp green pesto
- 225 ml soured cream
- The juice of ½ lemon
- 900 g chicken thighs, skin on (boneless)
- 450 g cauliflower

- 1 leek
- 3 tbsp butter
- 200 g grated cheddar cheese
- 120 g cherry tomatoes
- salt and pepper

Preparation:

1. Pre-heat oven to 200°C (400°F).
2. In a bowl, combine pesto, soured cream, and lemon juice. Season with salt and pepper and set aside.
3. Season thighs with salt and pepper. Place them in a 9 x 13" oven-proof frying pan on medium heat and fry on both sides until golden. Pour the cream mixture evenly over the chicken thighs.
4. Cut the tomatoes in bit-size pieces and chop the leak finely. Separate cauliflower into small florets. Add the veggies in an even layer on top of the cream mixture and chicken. Sprinkle the grated cheddar cheese on top.
5. Cover with aluminium foil and transfer to oven. Bake for 20 minutes and remove the foil. Bake for another 15 minutes or until the chicken is done. If the casserole is at risk of burning before it's done, cover it with a piece of aluminium foil, lower the heat and let cook for a little longer.

Mash and salsa verde pork skewers

....

Time: 15 minutes | Serves: 4
Net carbs: 7 g
Fibre: 5 g
Fat: 93 g
Protein: 30 g
Kcal: 956

Ingredients:

Pork skewers

- 500 g cubed pork shoulder
- 1 tsp pink Himalayan salt
- 1 tbsp butter
- ½ tbsp salt-free ranch seasoning
- **Cauliflower mash**

- 600 g cauliflower florets
- 60 g parmesan cheese (grated)
- 150 gbutter
- salt andpepper

Salsa Verde

- 50 gfresh cilantro (finely chopped)
- 100 g fresh parsley (finely chopped)
- 2 garlic cloves
- Juice of ½ lemon

- 150 ml olive oil
- 50 ml small capers
- 1 tsp pink Himalayan salt
- ½ tsp ground black pepper

Preparation:

1. **Pork Skewers:** Season the pork shoulder cubes with the ranch seasoning and pink Himalaya salt. Place the seasoned pork cubes on 8 wooden skewers. Place butter in a frying pan and heat on medium heat. Fry pork skewers for 2-3 minutes on each side until completely cooked. Remove from pan and set aside on a paper towel-lined plate.

2. **Cauliflower Mash:** Bring a pot with lightly salted water to a boil. Add the cauliflower florets and boil until cooked. Florets should be soft but still retain shape. Remove from water, drain, and pat dry the florets for a firmer mash. Add the florets, cheese, butter, and pepper to a food processor. Pulse to the desired consistency.

3. **Salsa Verde:** Place all salsa ingredients in a beaker. Use an immersion blender to mix the ingredients for 2 minutes.

4. Serve 2 pork skewers with ¼ of the cauliflower mash, and a drizzle of salsa Verde! Enjoy!

Salmon burgers with lemon butter and mash

Time: 25 minutes | Serves: 4
Net carbs: 7 g
Fibre: 3 g
Fat: 91 g
Protein: 45 g
Kcal: 1030

Ingredients:

Burgers

- 750 g salmon (cubed)
- 1 egg
- ½ yellow onion (medium)
- Salt and pepper
- 2 oz. butter, for frying

Broccoli Mash

- 500 gr broccoli florets
- 60ggrated parmesan cheese
- 140gbutter
- salt and pepper to taste

Lemonbutter

- 2 tbsp lemon juice
- 110 gr butter at room temperature
- salt and pepper to taste

Preparation:

1. **Salmon burgers:** Pre-heat oven to 100°C (220°F). Place the salmon, onion, egg and salt and pepper in a food processor. Pulse for half a minute into a coarse mixture. Do not overmix!
2. Form 8 burger patties. Placethe butter into a mediumfryingpan and heat over medium heat. Frythe burger patties for 5 minutes on each side. Place in the pre-heated oven to keep warm.
3. **Broccoli Mash:** Place water and a pinch of salt in a pot and bring to a boil. Add the broccoli and allow 2 minutes to cook until soft. Remove from water and drain.
4. Place the soften broccoli, butter, parmesan, and salt and pepper in a food processor. Pulse until a smooth paste is formed.

5. **Lemon Butter:** Use electric beaters tocombine the butter, lemon juice, and salt and pepper.
6. Place 2 burgers, ¼ of the broccoli mas, and ¼ of the melting lemon butter on a plate and enjoy!

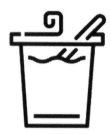

Fried chicken and roasted veggies

Time: 40 minutes | Serves: 2
Net carbs: 4.5 g
Fibre: 3 g
Fat: 41.5 g
Protein: 33.5 g
Kcal: 530

Ingredients:

Fried chicken

- ♦ 2 medium chicken breasts (boneless)
- ♦ 15 g butter, for frying
- ♦ 55 g herb butter, for serving

Roasted vegetables

- ♦ 230 g Brussels sprouts
- ♦ 110 gcherry tomatoes
- ♦ 110 g mushrooms
- ♦ Salt and pepper to taste
- ♦ ½ tsp dried rosemary
- ♦ 65 ml olive oil

Preparation:

1. **Fried chicken:** Place butter in a frying pan over medium heat. Season chicken breasts with salt and pepper and add to pan. Fry until internal temperature is 74°C (165°F). To check temperature use meat thermometer and insert half way into the largest chicken breast. Remove from pan and set aside.
2. **Roasted veggies:** Pre-heat oven to 200°C (400°F). In a bowl, mix the vegetables with olive oil and season with rosemary, salt, and pepper. Place the vegetables in a baking tray and bake for 20 minutes. The vegetables should be slightly caramelized.
3. Arrange one chicken breast and ¼ of the vegetables on each plate. Add the herb butter on the hot chicken and serve immediately! Enjoy!

Bacon and beef burger casserole

Time: 40 minutes | Serves: 2
Net carbs: 8 g
Fibre: 2 g
Fat: 91 g
Protein: 46 g
Kcal: 1041

Ingredients:

- 200 g diced smoked or unsmoked bacon
- 1 tbsp butter
- 400 g mince beef
- 2 chopped tomatoes
- 2 chopped dill pickles
- 1 garlic clove

- 2 eggs
- 2 tbsp concentrate tomato paste
- 200 g grated cheddar cheese
- 250 ml double cream
- salt and pepper

Preparation:

1. Pre-heat the oven to 200°C(400°F).
2. Heat the butter in an oven-proof frying panon moderate heat. Add the diced bacon and fry until golden. Increase heat and add themince beef. Stir to break the minceinto small pieces and fry until cooked through.
3. Lower the heat and add the chopped tomatoes anddill pickles. Incorporate the minced garlic into the mix along with two thirds of the cheese. Season with and salt and pepper.
4. In a bowl, mix the double cream, eggs, and tomato paste until combined. Season with salt and pepper and pour evenly on top of the beef mixture. Topthe pan with the remaining cheddar cheese.
5. Place the pan into thepre-heatedoven and bake for 20 minutes. The top layer should turn golden-brown.
6. Remove from oven and allow 10 minutes to rest. Arrange on plates and serve with freshly cut romaine lettuce drizzled with a touch of olive oil.

Broccoli and beef skillet

Time: 40 minutes | Serves: 2
Net carbs: 5 g
Fibre: 3 g
Fat: 54 g
Protein: 33 g
Kcal: 648

Ingredients:

- 275 g broccoli florets
- 300 g ground beef
- 75 g butter
- salt and pepper

Optional

- 125 ml crème fraîche or mayonnaise

Preparation:

1. Place a large frying pan over medium heat and add 25 grams of butter. Make sure both the beef and broccoli can fit in the pan.
2. Add the mince beef to the pan. Turn the heat on high and cook the beef until golden brown, but not entirely cooked through. Sprinkle salt and pepper to taste.
3. Reduce heat back to medium and add the broccoli and 25 more grams of butter. Cook the broccoli until cooked through (5 minutes). Season broccoli when done. Stir the mince beef occasionally while the broccoli cooks.
4. Add the remaining butter to the hot skillet with the remaining butter. Serve immediately with preferred side: mayonnaise or crème fraiche.

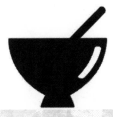

One-pot green beans and fried salmon

Time: 40 minutes | Serves: 2
Net carbs: 5 g
Fibre: 3 g
Fat: 58 g
Protein: 28 g
Kcal: 657

Ingredients:

- 2 x 125 g salmon steaks
- 300 g fresh green beans, rinsed and trimmed
- 100 g butter
- salt and pepper

Preparation:

1. Heata large frying pan on mediumhit andadd ⅔ of thebutter.
2. Add the green beans to the pan and allow to fry the green beans for 4 minutes. Sprinkle salt and pepper and move to one side of the pan.
3. Add a little more butter and place the two salmon steaks in the pan next to the beans. Fry the salmon on each side for 1-2 minutes. Stir the green beans occasionally while the salmon cooks. Season the salmon.
4. Remove from heat and arrange the salmon and green beans on plates. Serve with the butter.

TIP!

Substitute the green beans with zucchini, cauliflower, asparagus, broccoli or spinach.

Roasted veggie and cheese plate

Time: 40 minutes | Serves: 2
Net carbs: 9 g
Fibre: 6 g
Fat: 99 g
Protein: 21 g
Kcal: 1013

Ingredients:

- ½ zucchini
- ⅓ aubergine
- 60 ml olive oil
- Juice of ½ a lemon
- 10 black olives

- 150 g cheddar cheese or brie cheese
- 2 tbsp raw almonds
- 30 g leafy greens
- 125 ml crème fraiche
- salt and pepper

Preparation:

1. Pre-heat the oven to 225°C (450°F). Line a baking tray with baking sheet.
2. Cut the zucchini and aubergine lengthwise into ½-inch-thick slices. Season with salt on both sides and place on a paper-towel-lined plate. Set aside for 10minutes
3. Pat dry the zucchini and aubergine slices with clean paper towels. Place the slices on the baking tray and sprinkle with olive oil and ground pepper.
4. Allow 10 minutes to roast. Flip and allow 10 more minutes to roaston the other side. They should be golden-brown on both sides. Remove from oven.
5. Arrange aubergine and zucchini slices on serving platter. Add the cubed cheese, black olives, and greens (spinach, lettuce, rocket). Crush the almonds with a knife blade and sprinkle on the leafy greens. Drizzle lemon juice and olive oil over the roast veggies and serve with crème fraiche.

Minced lamb shepherd's pie

Time: 40 minutes | Serves: 2
Net carbs: 7 g
Fibre: 3 g
Fat: 98 g
Protein: 34 g
Kcal: 1042

Ingredients:

For the minced lamb:

- 800 g minced lamb meat (beef or pork)
- 1 tsp onion powder
- 2 tbsp tamari soy sauce
- 2 tbsp Worcestershire sauce
- ½ tbsp tabasco
- salt and pepper
- 1 tbsp butter, for frying

For the cauliflower mash:

- 650 g cauliflower florets
- 125 ml crème fraîche
- 75 g butter, melted
- 1 egg
- ½ finely chopped leek
- 150 g grated cheddar cheese
- salt and ground black pepper

Preparation:

1. **For the minced lamb:** Heat the butter on medium heat in an oven-proof medium frying pan. Add the minced lamp meat along with spices and tamari soy and Worcestershire sauces to the pan. Allow to fry until almost brown.
2. **For the mash:** Bring a pot of salted water to a gentle boil and add the cauliflower florets. Allow to cook until soft. Remove from pot, drain, and placeinto a food processor. Mash to desired consistency.
3. Incorporate the egg, finely chopped leek, butter, and crème fraîche into the mash. Add in half of the grated cheese and mix until well combined. Season to taste.

4. **Assemble the pie:** Spread the meat to form an even layer in the oven-proof pan. Top with even layers of mashed cauliflower and remaining cheese. Place in the oven and bake at 175°C (350°F) for 20-30 minutes until golden. Remove from oven and allow 10 minutes to rest.

5. Serve with leafy greens of choice! Enjoy!

Slow-cooked pulled pork with avocado humus

Time: 4h40 minutes | Serves: 2
Net carbs: 7 g
Fibre: 3 g
Fat: 98 g
Protein: 34 g
Kcal: 1042

Ingredients:

Avocado Humus

- 3 avocados, cut in halves and pitted
- Juice of ½ lemon
- fresh cilantro
- 60 ml olive oil
- 35 g sunflower seeds

- 2 tbsp tahini
- ½ tsp ground cumin
- 1 garlic clove
- salt and pepper

Pulled pork

- 900g pork shoulder
- 1 tbspcocoa powder
- ½ tbsp ground ginger
- ½ tbsp ground black pepper
- ½ tbsp paprika powder

- ½tsp cayenne pepper
- ½ tsp fennel seeds
- 2 tbsp olive oil
- 1 tbsp salt

Roasted tomato salad

- 500 g cherry tomatoes
- 1 tsp sea salt
- ground black pepper to taste
- 3 tbsp olive oil
- 2 finely chopped green onionsprings
- 1 tbspred wine vinegar

Preparation:

1. **Pulled pork:** Place the spices and olive oil in a small bowl and combine well. Rub the pork shoulder thoroughly with the mixture on all sides. Place the pork shoulder in a slow cooker. Allow 6 hours to cook on slow. Remove from the cooker. Shred the meat into small pieces using two forks.

2. **Avocado humus:** Place the avocado halves and all ingredients for the humus in a food processor. Mix until desired consistency. Thin the humous with water, lemon juice, or olive oil if too thick. Add salt and pepper to preference.

3. **Roasted tomato salad:** Mix the tomatoes, olive oil, and salt and pepper and spread on a baking paper-lined oven-proof pan. Roast for 15 minutes at 225°C (440°F). Turn off the heat and leave in the oven for 5-10more minutes. Remove from the oven. Sprinkle the green onions, olive oil, and vinegar.

4. Arrange the pulled pork, avocado humous, and roasted tomato salad on plates. Enjoy!

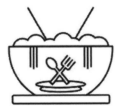

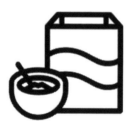

30-Day Keto Challenge

Whether you blame your hectic work schedule or your lack of inspiration and talent, you probably don't spend too much time in the kitchen. You, like so many other people, feel too tired to pick up groceries and make your own food. It's easier to stop at a take-out or just order something through an app. Well, it is time to stop this harmful behaviour because this 30-day challenge is really the ideal meal plan to get you started on your keto lifestyle that will render you slimmer, happier, and more energetic than ever!

Use the meal plan as a guideline. Adapt the ingredients and preparation methods to your personal preferences. Stick to the lowest carb intake that is sustainable on the long run for you and eat just enough fat that you feel great! As you complete each day of the challenge, you will become more aware of the actual nutrition packed in each food. You will learn to distinguish what makes you feel tired and what makes you feel fuller longer. You will learn what works for you and your body!

Your aim should not be to complete yet another diet challenge, but to adopt a new, healthier lifestyle. You should feel full quicker and have enough energy to work out more or, at least, consistently. Remember that the keto diet is not governed by a military-like discipline. It is flexible except when it comes to starches and sugars. Once you start feeling better without those elements, you will no longer crave them or want to try them!It is time to getcreative!

DAY 1

Breakfast

Low-carb mushroom omelette

Time: 15 minutes | Serves: 1
Net carbs: 4 g
Fibre: 1 g
Fat: 43 g
Protein: 25 g
Kcal: 510

Ingredients

- 3 free-range eggs
- 30 g grated cheddar cheese
- ⊠ yellow onion, julienned
- 3 mushrooms, trimmed and sliced
- salt and pepper
- 30 g butter, for frying

Preparation:

1. In a medium bowl, whisk the eggs with salt and pepper until frothy and smooth.
2. Place the butter in a non-stick frying pan on medium heat and allow to melt. Add the eggmixture and allow to cook until the omelette is set around the edges. The top should be still raw. Top it up with sliced mushrooms, grated cheese, and julienned onion on top.
3. Fold the omelette over in half with a spatula. Allow to cook for 1 minute until golden-brown on the bottom side. Flip and fry on the other side. Slideon to a plate and serve! Enjoy

Lunch

Bun-less Cheeseburgers (Page 22)

Dinner

Hearty Chicken Casserole (Page 36)

DAY 2

Breakfast
Cottage Cheese Pancakes with Berries (Page 10)

Lunch
Crispy Pancetta and Cauliflower Soup

Time: 25 minutes | Serves: 6
Net carbs: 6 g
Fibre: 3 g
Fat: 53 g
Protein: 10 g
Kcal: 534

Ingredients

- 1 litre chicken or vegetable broth
- 450 g finely sliced cauliflower (stems included)
- 1 tbsp Dijon mustard

- 200 g softcheese
- 100 g butter
- salt and pepper

Fried pancetta

- 200 g diced pancetta
- 1 tsp paprika powder

- 1 tbspbutter, for frying
- 75 g pecans

Preparation:

1. Pour the chicken or vegetable broth into a bot. Add the finely sliced cauliflower and allow to boil until soft. Remove from heat. Place the mixture into a food processor. Add the cheese, butter, and mustard and pulse to desired consistency. The longer blending, the smoother and creamier the soup. Season to taste!

2. Placea non-stick frying pan over medium heat and fry the diced pancetta in butter until crispy. Add the paprika powder and pecans when the pancetta is almost done. Remove from pan and set aside.

3. Place the cauliflower soup in bowls. Serve with pancetta mixture! Enjoy!

Dinner
Mash and Salsa Verde Pork Skewers (Page 37)

DAY 3

Breakfast
Classic bacon and eggs (Page 11)

Lunch
Keto Curried chicken wraps (page 23)

Dinner
Low-carb cod with roasted beets

Time: 50 minutes | Serves: 4
Net carbs: 9 g
Fibre: 3 g
Fat: 69 g
Protein: 46 g
Kcal: 852

Ingredients

- 3 tbsp butter, for frying
- 800 g cod code fillets

Roasted beets

- 450 g beets, peeled and cut into wedges
- 160 g blue cheese
- 3 tbsp olive oil
- salt and pepper
- 150 g herb butter

Preparation:

1. Preheat oven to 200°C 400°F (200°C).
2. Grease a baking tray and add the beet root edges. Top with crumbled cheese and olive oil. Season slightlyand place into the oven. Allow 25-30 minutes to cook. If the cheese has already browned, reduce heat and allow 5-10 minutes to cook until soften. Remove from oven and set aside

3. In a large frying pan, heat the butter. Add the cod fillets and fry to desired doneness. Season to taste. Remove from pan. Topthe fish with the herb butter and serve with roasted beets.

TIP!

Serve the fish with plenty of herb butter or pink herb butter.

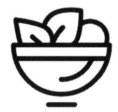

DAY 4

Breakfast
Bullet-proof coffee

Time: 5 minutes | Serves: 4
Net carbs: 6 g
Fibre: 3 g
Fat: 53 g
Protein: 10 g
Kcal: 534

Ingredients

- 2 tbsp unsalted butter
- 240 ml hot coffee
- 1 tbsp MCT oil

Preparation:

1. Add ingredients to a blender and mix until frothy and smooth.
2. Enjoy!

Lunch
Pesto salmon (Page 24)

Dinner
Salmon burgers with lemon butter and mash (Page 39)

DAY 5

Breakfast

Buttery coconut flour waffles (Page 12)

Lunch

Garam masala chicken

Time: 5 minutes | Serves: 4
Net carbs: 6 g
Fibre: 4 g
Fat: 51 g
Protein: 38 g
Kcal: 629

Ingredients

- 4 tbsp garam masala mix
- 650 g chicken breasts cut lengthwise
- 3 tbsp butter
- salt
- 1 finely sliced red bell pepper
- 300 ml double cream
- 1 tbsp finely chopped fresh parsley

Preparation:

1. Pre-heat the oven to 200°C (400°F).
2. Heat butter over moderate heat in a large, oven-proof frying pan. Fry on both sides until golden-brown. Add ½ of the garam masala mix. Stir to combine. Season with salt and pepper.
3. In a small bowl, mix the double cream with the sliced bell peppers and garam masala mix. Pour the mixture over the chicken breasts and placein the pre-heated oven. Allow 20 minutes to cook. Remove from oven and allow 10 minutes to cool.
4. Serve with chopped fresh parsley! Enjoy!

Dinner

Fried chicken and roasted veggies (page 41)

DAY 6

Breakfast
Buttery coconut flour waffles

Lunch
Cream-cheese keto turkey (page 25)

Dinner
Tandoori salmon with crunchy salad and cucumber sauce

Time: 5 minutes | Serves: 4
Net carbs: 8 g
Fibre: 9 g
Fat: 73 g
Protein: 35 g
Kcal: 847

Ingredients

- 2 tbsp olive oil
- 600 g salmon fillets

- 2 tbsp tandoori seasoning

Crunchy Salad

- 150 g rocket leaves
- 1 finely diced orange bell pepper
- 3 finely sliced green onion springs

- 4 cubed avocado halves
- Juice of 1 lime

Creamy cucumber sauce

- 175 ml soured cream
- ½ English cucumber, grated and drained
- 2 minced garlic cloves
- Juice of ½ lime

- Salt to taste

Preparation:

1. Pre-heat the oven to 175°C (350°F). line an oven-proof pan with baking paper. Ste aside.
2. **Salmon:** In a medium size bowl, mix the olive oil with tandoori seasoning. Add the salmon fillets and rub the fillets with the mixture on all sides. Arrange in pan and bake in oven for 20 minutes.Use a fork to check for doneness. Salmon should flake easily when done.
3. **Salad:** Combine rocket leaves, diced bell pepper, sliced spring onions, avocado cubes, and lime juice. Arrange on plates.
4. **Cucumber salad:** In a small bowl, mix grated cucumber, minced garlic, soured cream, and lime juice. Season to taste. Set aside.
5. **Assemble:** Place salmon fillets on plates next to the crispy salad. Spoon the cucumber sauce on top. Enjoy!

DAY 7

Breakfast

Tweaked scrambled eggs

Time: 5 minutes | Serves: 4
Net carbs: 2 g
Fibre: 1 g
Fat: 18 g
Protein: 14 g
Kcal: 229

Ingredients

- 6 free-range eggs
- 2 finely chopped pickled jalapeños
- 1 spring onion
- 1 finely chopped tomato
- 70 g grated cheddar cheese
- salt and pepper
- 2 tbsp butter, for frying

Preparation:

1. Heat the butter on medium heat in a non-stick frying pan. Add the chopped jalapenos, tomato, and spring onion. Fryfor 3 minutes.
2. Meanwhile, crack eggsin a small bowl and whisk until smooth andfrothy. Add whisked eggs over the sautéed vegetables. Use a spatula to scramble for 1-2 minutes. When done, incorporate grated cheese and season to taste.
3. **Serving suggestion:** Serve with romaine lettuce and avocado salad with a drizzle of vinaigrette dressing!

Lunch

Creamy cabbage with fried chorizo (page 26)

Dinner

Bacon and beef burger casserole (Page 42)

DAY 8

Breakfast
15-min creamy seafood omelette (page 13)

Lunch
Keto cabbage stir-fry (page 26)

Time: 5 minutes | Serves: 4
Net carbs: 10 g
Fibre: 5 g
Fat: 97 g
Protein: 31 g
Kcal: 1040

Ingredients

- 150 g butter
- 750 g shredded green cabbage
- 600 g mince pork
- 1 tsp salt
- 1 tsponion powder
- ¼ tsp ground black pepper

- 1 tbspred curry paste
- 1tbsp white winevinegar
- 2 garlic cloves
- fresh cilantro, finely chopped
- ½ finely chopped yellow onion,
- 240 ml soured cream or crème fraiche

Preparation:

1. Heat ½ butter in a workor large skillet over moderate-high heat. Add the shredded cabbage and sauté for 5 minutes or untilsoftened.
2. Stir in the white wine vinegar and spices (salt, onion powder, black pepper).Continue to cook until fragrant. Remove sautéed cabbage from wok and set aside.
3. In the same wok, add remaining butter. Allow to melt and stir in the minced garlic, curry paste, and chopped onion. Sauté for 1 minute. Add the minced meat and fry until cooked through stirring occasionally. Most of the liquid should have evaporated.
4. Reduce heat and return the cabbage to the wok. Stir to combine until warmed through. Season with salt and pepper and sprinkle chopped fresh coriander on top.

5.   Serving with soured cream.

Dinner
Broccoli and beef skillet (page 43)

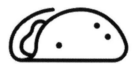

DAY 9

Breakfast

Guacamole and bacon breakfast tacos (page 15)

Lunch

Avocado and green beans pork chops (page 27)

Dinner

Herb butter fried chicken with leafy greens (page 41)

Time: 30 minutes | Serves: 4
Net carbs: 2 g
Fibre: 2 g
Fat: 64 g
Protein: 63 g
Kcal: 841

Ingredients

- Herb butter
- 150 g salted butter, at room temperature
- ½ tsp garlic powder
- 1 minced garlic clove
- 1 tsp lemon juice
- Chopped fresh parsley

Fried chicken

- 30 g butter, for frying
- 4 medium chicken breasts
- salt and pepper to taste

Leafy greens

- 225 g leafy greens of choice

Preparation:

1. **Herb Butter:** In a small bowl, combine all the ingredients for herb butter. Use parsley to suit personal preference. Set aside.

2. **Fried Chicken:** Season to taste the chicken breasts. Heat the butter in a large frying pan over moderate heat. Add the chicken breasts and fry on both sides until cooked through. When done, the inner temperature of the largest chicken breast should be 75° (165°F).

3. **Assembling:** Arrange the leafy greens of choice on each plate. Place chicken breast over the bed of greens and top with the herb butter. Serve immediately! Enjoy!

DAY 10

Breakfast
Mayo and boiled eggs

Time: 10 minutes | Serves: 2
Net carbs: 1 g
Fibre: 0 g
Fat: 29 g
Protein: 11 g
Kcal: 316

Ingredients

- ♦ 4 eggs
- ♦ 4 tbsp mayonnaise

Preparation:

1. Bring water to a boil in apot. Carefully, place the eggsin the water. Boil the eggs for 5–6 minutes for soft-boiled eggs, 6–8 minutes for medium and 8–10 minutes for hard-boiled eggs.
2. Serve with mayonnaise.

TIP!

Serve with sautéed asparagus or sliced avocado!

Lunch
Kale and pork with fried eggs (page 28)

Dinner
One-pot fried green and salmon (page 44)

DAY 11

Breakfast
Brussel sprouts hash (page 16)

Lunch
Fried salmon and Asian-style cabbage

Time: 20 minutes | Serves: 4
Net carbs: 11 g
Fibre: 7 g
Fat: 96 g
Protein: 41 g
Kcal: 1093

Ingredients

Asian-style cabbage

- 800 g finely sliced green cabbage
- 2 tbsp coconut oil
- 1 tbsp sesame oil

- 1 tbsp red curry paste
- salt and pepper

Fried salmon

- 90 g butter
- 750 g salmon fillets
- 20 g sesame seeds

- salt and pepper
- 240 ml mayonnaise for serving

Preparation:

1. **Curried cabbage:** Add coconut oil to a wok and heat over high heat. Add in the finely sliced cabbage and stir to coat. Add the curry paste and stir until combined. Allow to sauté until golden but stillcrispy.Season with salt and pepper and stirin the sesame oil. Mix thoroughly. Remove from heat and keep hot until serving.

2. **Fried salmon:** Heat the butter in a medium-size frying pan over fairly high heat. Season the salmon fillets with salt and pepper. Coat with sesame seeds on all sides. Fry the salmon fillets on each side for 2 minutes while occasionally basting the fillets with the melted butter. Remove salmon from pan. Reserve the melted butter.

3. Arrange the salmon fillets on plates. Drizzle with the sautéed butter and serve with the Asian-style cabbage, lime wedges, and mayo. Enjoy!

Dinner
Roasted veggies and cheese plate (page 45)

DAY 12

Breakfast

Keto oatmeal (page 17)

Lunch

Roasted bell peppers and fried halloumi cheese (page 29)

Dinner

Fried pork chops with cheese sauce

Time: 5 minutes | Serves: 4
Net carbs: 4 g
Fibre: 1 g
Fat: 64 g
Protein: 61 g
Kcal: 849

Ingredients

- 2 tbsp unsalted butter, for frying
- 4 pork chops, seasoned with salt and pepper
- 175 ml double cream, crumbled
- 150 g blue Stilton cheese or Gorgonzola cheese
- 1 tbsp unsalted butter
- 250 g green beans, fresh, trimmed and rinsed

Preparation:

1. **Cheese sauce:** Add double cream to a medium size frying pan on medium heat. Bring to agentle simmer. When the double cream has started simmering, add the crumbled blue cheese.
2. Increase heat to medium. Stir gently while simmeringfor 1-2 minutes until the sauce has thickened to a creamy consistency. The sauce should coat the spatula evenly when done. Remove from heat and set aside.

3. **Pork chops:** Placebutter in a medium frying panon medium-high heat. Allow to melt and add the pork chops. Fry for 2-3 minutes on each side. When done, the internal temperature of thickest pork chop should be 63°-71°C (145°-160°F). Remove from pan and place in an airtight container for3 minutes.

4. **Fried green beans:** Heat butter in a medium frying pan on moderate heat. Add the green beans and fry for 3-5 minutes to desired doneness. Seasonthe beans with salt and freshly ground black pepper!

5. **Assemble:** Place the pork chops on a bed of fried green beans. Topwith a generous amount ofblue cheese sauce! Serve immediately! Enjoy!

TIP!

Mix the juices from the pan where you fried the pork chops into the cheese sauce. Re-heat the sauce if necessary!

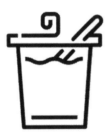

DAY 13

Breakfast
Chorizo and spring onion muffin

Time: 25 minutes | Serves: 6
Net carbs: 2 g
Fibre: 0 g
Fat: 26 g
Protein: 23 g
Kcal: 336

Ingredients

- 1-2 green onion springs, finely chopped
- 150 g chorizo sausage, diced
- 12 free-range eggs
- 175 g grated cheese
- salt and pepper

Preparation:

1. Heat oven to 175°C (350°F).
2. Place non-stick baking cups in a 12-cup muffin tray or grease a non-stick muffin tray.
3. Mix diced chorizo and sliced green onions. Place some of the mixture to the bottom of each cup of the muffin tray.
4. Whisk eggs until smooth and frothy. Stir in cheese, preferably blue cheese. Season with freshly ground pepper and salt, only if the cheese is not already salty.
5. Pour the egg and cheese mixture over the chorizo and scallions.Place in oven and bake for 15 minutes. Leave longer if the muffin tray has taller cups.
6. Remove from oven! Serve immediately.

Lunch
Cloud bread BLT (page 30)

Dinner
Minced lamb shepherd's pie (page 46)

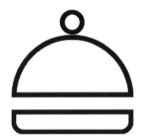

DAY 14

Breakfast

Keto turkey and avocado plate (page 17)

Lunch

Fried lamb with herbed butter

Time: 40 minutes | Serves: 4
Net carbs: 0.3 g
Fibre: 0 g
Fat: 62 g
Protein: 43 g
Kcal: 729

Ingredients

- 1 tbsp butter
- 1 tbsp olive oil
- 8 lamb chops, at room temperature
- salt and pepper

Preparation:

1. Make several cuts into the fat of the lamb chops to prevent curling up when cooked. Make sure to cut all through the more resistant fat. Salt and pepper the chops to preference.
2. Heat the butter and oil into amedium frying pan on moderate heat. Add the lamb chops and fry for 3-4 minutes on each side depending desired doneness and the thickness of the chops.
3. Transfer chops to plates and top with a generous amount of herbed butter. Serve with lemon wedges! Enjoy!

Dinner

Slow-cooked pulled pork with avocado humous (page 48)

DAY 15

Breakfast
Spinach frittata keto style (page 19)

Lunch
Asian-style sesame fried beef salad (page 32)

Dinner
Chinese pork with fried green cabbage

Time: 120 minutes | Serves: 4
Net carbs: 6 g
Fibre: 5 g
Fat: 117 g
Protein: 22 g
Kcal: 1178

Ingredients

Fried cabbage

- 50 gr unsalted butter
- 600 g green cabbage, chopped coarsely
- 2 crushed garlic cloves
- 1 tsp Szechuan pepper
- 1 tbsp rice vinegar
- salt and pepper

Chinese pork

- 800 g pork belly
- 1 tbsp five spice mix
- 1 tbsp rice vinegar
- 1 tsp salt
- 75 ml coarse salt to coat

Preparation:

1. **Fried green cabbage:** Heat butter on mediumheat in a large non-stick frying pan. Add the crushed garlic andcabbage. Fry while stirring frequently until golden-brown. When almost done, stir in the rice vinegar and seasonings. Remove from heat and set aside!

2. **Chinese pork:** Gently pat the meat dry with paper towels. Skin side up on a cutting board, score the skin (only the skin, not the fat) finely with a sharp knife. Mix the vinegar and seasonings and brush them into the meat. Do not brush the skin!

3. Create a tray-like package out of aluminium foil and place the meat inside. Place the package in a baking tray in the fridge for 12 hours for the meat to dry and become crispy when cooked.

4. Pre-heat oven to 200°C (400°F). Remove the pork belly from fridge and cover the skin with an even and generous layer of coarse salt. Place on the lowest rack in the oven and let roast for 60 minutes. Inner temperature should read 80°C (160°F).

5. Remove from oven. Remove the pork belly from the aluminium foil package. Reserve the juices and rendered fat. Scrape the coarse salt off the skin. Return pork belly to oven tray and place in oven under the broiler.

6. Let broil for 20 or 30 minutes. The skin should be bubbly, crisp, and golden brown when done. Remove from oven. Set aside to cool down for 5 minutes. Slice the pork belly to desired thickness and serve on a bed offried green cabbage. Serve immediately! Enjoy!

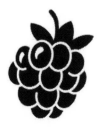

DAY 16

Breakfast

Ketogenic porridge

Time: 10 minutes | Serves: 1
Net carbs: 4 g
Fibre: 5 g
Fat: 64 g
Protein: 12 g
Kcal: 642

Ingredients

- 12 g sesame seeds
- 12 g chia seeds
- 1 free-range egg
- 75 ml double cream
- salt
- 30 g coconut oil or butter, for frying
- Raspberry jam, for serving

Preparation:

1. Whisk the eggs until frothy and smooth. Add all ingredients except butter and mix to combine. Set aside.
2. Heat coconut oil or butter in a non-stick pan over moderate heat.
3. Add the egg mixture to the pan and allow to thicken while stirring. Allow the porridge to simmer. Do not let it boil.
4. Remove from heat! Serve the porridge while hot with immediately with raspberry jam.

Lunch

Bun-less cheeseburgers (page 22)

Dinner

Hearty chicken casserole (page 36)

DAY 17

Breakfast
Cottage cheese pancakes with berries (page 10)

Lunch
Crab and red cheese casserole

Time: 40 minutes | Serves: 4
Net carbs: 5 g
Fibre: 2 g
Fat: 91 g
Protein: 47 g
Kcal: 1038

Ingredients

- 30 g butter, for frying
- 150 g celery stalks, finely chopped
- 1 medium yellow onion, finely chopped
- 300 ml crème fraiche or soured cream
- 4 free-range eggs
- 300 g grated red cheddar

- 480 g crab meat (canned, drained)
- ¼ tsp cayenne pepper
- 2 tsp paprika powder
- salt and pepper
- 80 gr leafy greens
- 2 tbsp olive oil

Preparation:

1. Heat oven to 200°C (400°F).
2. Heat butter in a medium frying pan. Add celery and onion and fry until translucent. Season to taste. Remove from heat and set aside.
3. In a medium-size salad bowl, mix crème fraiche, crab meat, eggs, and ⅔ of the shredded cheese. Stir in the fried celery and onion and seasonings.
4. Grease a baking dish and spread the mixture evenly on the bottom. Top with remaining cheese andallow to bakeuntil the cheesebecomes golden-brown (20 minutes). Remove from oven and allow 5 minutes to rest.
5. Mix leafy greens of choice with olive oil. Serve with the crab meat and cheese casserole.

Dinner
Mash and salsa verde pork skewers (page 37)

DAY 18

Breakfast

Buttery coconut flour waffles (page 12)

Lunch

Curried chicken wraps (page 23)

Dinner

Chicken a la Provence

Time: 75 minutes | Serves: 4
Net carbs: 5 g
Fibre: 3 g
Fat: 78 g
Protein: 43 g
Kcal: 911

Ingredients

- 900 g boneless, skin-on chicken thighs
- 4 finely sliced garlic cloves
- 125 ml pitted black olives
- 250 g cherry tomatoes

- 60 ml olive oil
- 1 tbsp dried oregano
- salt and pepper

Mayo Lettuce Salad

- 200 g lettuce, coarsely chopped
- Zest of ¼ lemon
- 225 ml mayonnaise

- 1 tsp paprika powder
- salt and pepper

Preparation:

1. Heat oven to 200°C (400°F).

2. **Chicken thighs:** Arrange the chicken thighs side up on a baking tray. Place the olives, sliced garlic, and cherry tomatoes around the thighs. Drizzle olive oil on top. Season with salt andpepper and driedoregano.

3. Place the thighs in the oven and let roast until cooked through. Chicken thighs are done in 45-60 minutes or when inner temperature in the thickest thigh reads 75°C (180°F). Remove from oven and set aside until ready to serve!

4. **Mayo lettuce salad:** Mix the salad ingredients until the lettuce is evenly coated with the mayo and seasonings, including lemon zest.

5. Place the chicken thighs on a bed of mayo lettuce salad. Serve immediately! Enjoy!

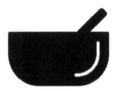

DAY 19

Breakfast
Mackerel in tomato sauce and egg breakfast

Time: 5 minutes | Serves: 2
Net carbs: 4 g
Fibre: 1 g
Fat: 59 g
Protein: 35 g
Kcal: 689

Ingredients

- 2 tbsp butter for frying
- 225 g mackerel in tomato sauce, canned
- 4 free-range eggs
- ½ red onion, julienned
- 50 g lettuce, chopped coarsley
- 60 ml olive oil
- salt and pepper

Preparation:

1. Place butter in a medium pan over moderate heat. Allow to melt. Crack eggs and fry to preference.
2. Mix lettuce red onion, and olive oil. Season to taste.
3. **Assemble:** Place salad, mackerel, and eggs on plates. Enjoy!

Lunch
Fried chicken and roasted veggies (page 41)

Dinner
Pesto salmon (page 24)

DAY 20

Breakfast
15-min creamy seafood omelette (page 13)

Lunch
One-pot fried mushrooms and halloumi cheese

Time: 15 minutes | Serves: 2
Net carbs: 7 g
Fibre: 2 g
Fat: 74 g
Protein: 36 g
Kcal: 830

Ingredients

- 75 g butter
- 300 g grilling cheese, preferably halloumi
- 300 g mushrooms, trimmed and quartered

- 10 green olives
- salt and pepper

Optional

- 125 ml crème fraiche, soured cream or mayonnaise

Preparation:

1. In a medium frying pan, heat the butter. Add the mushroom quarters and let fry for 4 minutes. They should look nice and golden. Season with salt and pepper.
2. Move the mushrooms to one side of the pan. Add the halloumi slices and fry on each side for 2 minutes. Occasionally stir the mushrooms.
3. Place mushrooms, grilled cheese and green olives on a plate. Serve with crème fraiche, soured cream or mayonnaise!

Dinner

Salmon burgers with lemon butter and mash (page 39)

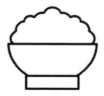

DAY 21

Breakfast
Smoked salmon and scrambled eggs sandwich (page 14)

Lunch
Cream cheese keto turkey (page 25)

Dinner
Goat cheese courgette boats

Time: 5 minutes | Serves: 2
Net carbs: 5 g
Fibre: 2 g
Fat: 62 g
Protein: 27 g
Kcal: 693

Ingredients

- 4 tbsp olive oil
- 1 large courgette
- 2 finely sliced garlic cloves
- 50 g baby spinach
- salt and pepper to taste
- 2tbsp marinara sauce, divided
- 200 g goat cheese, crumbled
- Freshly chopped parsley

Preparation:

1. Preheat oven to 375°F(190°C).
2. **Prepare the boats:** Cut the courgette in half lengthwise. Spoon out the seeds and reserve. Place the courgette halves in an oven-proof pan.
3. Heat ½ of the oil in a medium frying pan on moderate heat. Add the garlic and let fry until fragrant. Add the spinach and courgette seeds. Allow to fry stirring occasionally until softened. Season with salt and pepper.

4. **Assemble the boats:** spoon the marinara sauce on top of the courgette halves. Add an even layer of the spinach and garlic mixture. Add the crumbled goat cheese on top of each courgette boat.

5. Place the courgette halves/boats in the oven and let bake for 25-35 minutes to desired tenderness. The cheese should have a nice goldencolour. Remove from oven and let rest for a couple of minutes.

6. **Serving:** Place the courgette boatson plates and drizzle with remaining olive oil. Garnishwith freshly chopped parsley. Season with a little more pepper! Enjoy!

DAY 22

Breakfast
Smoked salmon stuffed avocados

Time: 5 minutes | Serves: 4
Net carbs: 6 g
Fibre: 13 g
Fat: 71 g
Protein: 58 g
Kcal: 911

Ingredients

- 180 g smoked salmon
- 2 avocados, halvedand pitted
- 150 ml crème fraiche
- salt and pepper

Optional

- 2 tbsp lemon juice

Preparation:

1. Place avocado halves on plates. Spoon a generous amount of crème fraiche on top. Fold in smoked lemon slices and add over the crème fraiche.
2. Season with salt and pepper to taste.

TIP!

Squeeze a bit of lemon juiceover the avocados for a lemony flavour and to keep from turning brown! Substitute crème fraiche with mayonnaise or soured cream.

Lunch
Creamy cabbage with fried chorizo (page 26)

Dinner

Bacon and beef burger casserole (page 42)

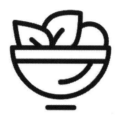

DAY 23

Breakfast

Guacamole and bacon breakfast tacos (page 15)

Lunch

Ketogenic Cobb salad

Time: 10 minutes | Serves: 2
Net carbs: 7 g
Fibre: 8 g
Fat: 97 g
Protein: 61 g
Kcal: 1161

Ingredients

- 75 g diced smoked bacon
- ½ whole roast chicken
- 2 free-range
- 50 g blue cheese, crumbled
- 1 avocado, halved, pitted, and diced

- 1 large tomato, finely sliced
- 150 g Romaine lettuce, chopped coarsely
- salt and ground black pepper
- Optional:
- Finely sliced fresh chives

Mayo dressing

- 1 tbsp ranch seasoning
- 3 tbsp mayonnaise

- 2 tbspwater
- salt andground black pepper

Preparation:

1. **Dressing:** In a small bowl, place all dressing ingredients and mix until combined. Set aside.
2. **Eggs:** Bring a pot of salted water to a boil. Gently lower the eggs and boil to preference. Remove from boiling water and place in iced-water. Peel and chop roughly.
3. **Bacon and chicken:** heat a small frying pan on moderate heat. Add bacon and fry until crispy. Shred the rotisserie chicken with two forks.
4. On a large plate, mix lettuce, avocado, and tomato. Season with salt and pepper.

5. Distribute the crispy bacon and shredded chicken evenly on the veggie bed. Sprinkle the crumbled cheese and shopped eggs on top. Drizzle with the mayo dressing and garnish with finely chopped chives. Enjoy!

Dinner
Broccoli and beef skillet (page 43)

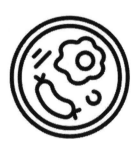

DAY 24

Breakfast
Brussel sprouts hash (page 16)

Lunch
Avocado and green beans pork chops (page 27)

Dinner
Fried pork belly with tender Brussel sprouts

Time: 40 minutes | Serves: 4

Net carbs: 7 g

Fibre: 5 g

Fat: 97 g

Protein: 19 g

Kcal: 993

Ingredients

- 550 g pork belly cut to bite-sized pieces
- 450 gBrussels sprouts, trimmed, and halved
- 2crushed garlic cloves
- 75 g butter
- 1 tbsp rice vinegar
- 2 tbsp dark soy sauce
- ½ finely sliced leek
- salt and ground black pepper

Preparation:

1. Heat a medium size frying pan on moderate heat. Add the pork belly pieces and increase heat. Fry until the pork belly becomes golden. Lower heat.
2. Add the smashed garlic, butter, and Brussel sprouts halves. Stir in and fry until golden-brown.
3. Add rice vinegar and dark soy and stir to combine. Season with salt and pepper. Add the leeks and gently combine with the pork and Brussel sprouts hash. Remove from heat. Serve immediately!

DAY 25

Breakfast

Breakfast tuna salad

Time: 5 minutes | Serves: 4
Net carbs: 1 g
Fibre: 0 g
Fat: 26 g
Protein: 8 g
Kcal: 271

Ingredients

- 120 g tuna in olive oil, drained
- 100 ml mayonnaise
- 2 tbsp full-fat soured cream or crème fraiche
- 2 pickled cucumbers, diced
- ½ finely diced red onion
- salt and pepper
- ½ tsp chili flakes
- Chopped fresh parsley

Preparation:

1. Place all ingredients in a medium bowl and mix until combined well.
2. Serve the salad on low-carb bread or crispbread and eggs boiled to preference! Enjoy!

Lunch

Kale and pork with fried eggs (page 28)

Dinner

One-pot fried green beans and salmon (page 44)

DAY 26

Breakfast
Keto oatmeal (page 17)

Lunch
Spicy prawn and avocado salad

Time: 10 minutes | Serves: 4
Net carbs: 9 g
Fibre: 16 g
Fat: 79 g
Protein: 26 g
Kcal: 871

Ingredients

- 2 avocados, halved and pitted
- Juice of ½ lime
- 150 gcucumber, peeled and finely sliced
- 50 g baby spinach
- 3tbsp olive oil, for frying

- 280 g cooked and peeled prawns
- 2 tsp chili powder
- 275 g shrimp, peeled
- fresh cilantro, for serving

Dressing

- 60 ml olive oil
- 1 tbsp minced ginger
- ½ pressed garlic clove

- Juice of ½ lime
- ½ tbsp darksoy sauce
- salt and pepper, to taste

Preparation:

1. Cut avocado to desired size. Place in a bowl and add sliced cucumber, spinach, and lemon juice. Season with salt and pepper and mix to combine.
2. Heat oil in a small frying pan on moderate heat. Add chilli and garlic and fry until fragrant. Addthe cooked prawns and let warm a little. Season with salt and pepper. Stir to combine. Remove from heat.

3. Transfer the spicy prawns to the avocado bowl. Sprinkle freshly chopped coriander or parsley to taste.
4. Place all dressing ingredients into a food processor and pulse to combine. Drizzle the dressing over the avocado and shrimp salad.

TIP!

_____

Sprinkle some crushed nuts on top of the salad!

Dinner
Roasted veggies and cheese plate (page 45)

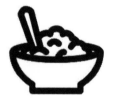

DAY 27

Breakfast
Keto turkey and avocado plate (page 17)

Lunch
Roasted bell peppers and fried halloumi cheese (page 29)

Dinner
Keto mussels' plate

Time: 10 minutes | Serves: 2
Net carbs: 7 g
Fibre: 14 g
Fat: 96 g
Protein: 34 g
Kcal: 1055

Ingredients

- 4 free-range eggs
- 240 g ready-to-eat mussels, divided
- 2 avocados, halved and pitted
- 50 g leafy greens chopped to desired size
- 125 ml mayonnaise

- 2 tbsp olive oil
- **Optional:**
- 110 g cottage cheese
- chopped fresh chives
- salt and pepper

Preparation:

1. **Eggs:** Place eggs gently into a pot of boiling water. Boil for 4 minutes for hard-boiled eggs and 8 minutes for soft eggs. Remove eggs from boiling water and cool in iced-cold water for 2 minutes. Remove the shell and cut in halves.
2. **Assemble plate:** Place egg, avocado, mayo, mussels, and olive-oil drizzled leafy greens plates. Serve with cottage cheese sprinkled with fresh chives and a touch of salt and pepper! Enjoy!

DAY 28

Breakfast
Buttery Gouda roll-ups

Time: 5 minutes | Serves: 4
Net carbs: 2 g
Fibre: 0 g
Fat: 31 g
Protein: 13 g
Kcal: 330

Ingredients

- 60 gbutter, room temperature
- 240 g gouda cheese, slices
- Paprika to taste
- Salt and pepper to taste

Preparation:

1. Arrange all goudacheese slices on acutting board. Spreadbutter on eachslice. Roll up! Enjoy!

TIPS!

Add paprika powder, chopped parsley, dried herbs, or chilli flakes to the butter to add extra flavour.

Lunch
Cloud bread BLT (page 30)

Dinner
Minced lamb shepherd's pie (page 46)

DAY 29

Breakfast
Spinach frittata keto style (page 19)

Lunch
Mexican "Buddha" bowl

Time: 5 minutes | Serves: 4
Net carbs: 9 g
Fibre: 11 g
Fat: 71 g
Protein: 41 g
Kcal: 862

Ingredients

- 75 g butter
- 700 g boneless, skin-on chicken thighs,cut into thin strips
- salt and pepper
- 2 tbsp fajita seasoning mix
- 1 yellow onion, julienned
- 1 green bell pepper, julienned
- 150 g plum cherry tomatoes, halved
- 250 g Romaine lettuce, chopped to preference
- 2 avocados, halved and pitted, diced
- 150 g grated Mexicancheese (or cheese of choice)
- Chopped fresh coriander (or parsley)

Preparation:

1. Heat butter in a medium sizefrying pan over moderate heat. Add chicken strips and fry until almost cooked through. Add salt and pepper and fajita seasoning. Stir to combine.
2. Add onion and pepper and allow to simmer until the veggies have softened, and the chicken has cooked through. Remove from heat and set aside.
3. Add lettuce to a salad bowl. Add the chicken strips on top. Place avocado, grated cheese, and tomatoes over the chicken like in a Buddha bowl.
4. Serve with a dollop of crème fraiche and chopped fresh parsley or coriander.

Dinner
Slow-cooked pulled pork with avocado humous (page 48)

DAY 30

Breakfast

Classic bacon and eggs (page 11)

Lunch

Asian-style sesame fried beef salad (page 32)

Dinner

Cheesy chicken with nutty salad

Time: 60 minutes | Serves: 4
Net carbs: 8 g
Fibre: 3 g
Fat: 76 g
Protein: 41 g
Kcal: 897

Ingredients

Nutty Salad

- 250 g romaine lettuce, chopped coarsely
- 100 g cherry tomatoes, cut in halves
- 2 tbsp olive oil
- 75 g nuts of choice (walnuts, pecans, almonds)

Cheesy chicken

- 50 g butter, for frying, divided
- 1 finely sliced medium leek
- 600 g boneless, skin-on chicken thighs
- 50 ml white wine
- 300 ml crème fraiche or soured cream
- 150 g blue cheese, preferably Stilton or Gorgonzola
- salt and pepper, to taste
- freshly chopped parsley

Preparation:

1. Pre-heat oven to 175°C (350°F).
2. **Nutty salad:** Mix lettuce and cherry tomato halves in a salad bowl. Drizzle with olive oil and sprinkle with the nuts of choice. Set aside.
3. **Leeks:** Heat ½ the butter in an oven-proof frying pan over moderate heat. Add the finely sliced leek and fry until softened. Season with sold and pepper and give it another stir. Spread the fried leeks evenly on the bottom of the pan.
4. **Chicken thighs:** In a separate pan, heat remaining butter and add chicken. Fry on both sides until golden. Transfer thighs on top of the bed of sautéed leeks in the oven-proof pan. Set aside.
5. **Cheesy sauce:** mix wine and crème fraiche in a medium sauce pan over medium heat. Bring to a gentle boil and let simmer for 2 minutes. Add the crumbled blue cheese and allow to melt stirring occasionally. Season with salt and pepper.
6. **Assemble:** Transfer the cheesy sauce on top of the fried chicken thighs. Place the pan in the oven until the chicken is cooked through. Inner temperature should read 72°C (161°F), which should take 15-20 minutes.
7. **Serving:** Remove from oven and allow 5 minutes to rest. Transfer to plates and enjoy wit freshly chopped parsley on top and nutty salad on the side!

EXCLUSIVE BONUS!

Get Keto Audiobook for FREE NOW!*

*The Ultimate Keto Diet Guide 2019-2020:
How to Loose weight with Quick and Easy Steps*

SCAN ME

or go to

www.free-keto.co.uk

*Listen free for 30 Days on Audible (for new members only)

Disclaimer

This book contains opinions and ideas of the author and is meant to teach the reader informative and helpful knowledge while being entertaining. The instructions and strategies are possibly not right for every reader and there is no guarantee that they work for everyone. Using this book and implementing the information / recipes therein contained is explicitly your own responsibility and risk. This work with all its contents, does not guarantee correctness, completion, quality or correctness of the provided information. Misinformation or misprints cannot be completely eliminated.

Legal notice

Printed in Great Britain
by Amazon

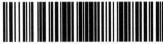

35654212R00064